The AIDS Awareness Library

When Someone You Know Has AIDS

Anna Forbes, MSS

The Rosen Publishing Group's
PowerKids Press
New York

Published in 1996 by The Rosen Publishing Group, Inc.
29 East 21st Street, New York, NY 10010

Copyright © 1996 by The Rosen Publishing Group, Inc.

All rights reserved. No part of this book may be reproduced in any form without permission in writing from the publisher, except by a reviewer.

First Edition

Photo credits: Cover © Jeff Greenberg/International Stock; p. 4 © George Ancona/International Stock; p. 7 © Stan Ries/International Stock; p. 8 © Mark Bolster/International Stock; p. 11 © Alain McLaughlin/Impact Visuals; p. 12 © Paul Avis/Liaison International; p. 15 © Jack Kurtz/Impact Visuals; p. 16 © Tom McKitterick/Impact Visuals; p. 19 © Yvonne Hemsey/Liaison International; p. 20 © Rick Reinhard/Impact Visuals.

Book Design and Layout: Erin McKenna

Forbes, Anna, MSS
    When someone you know has AIDS / Anna Forbes.
        p.   cm. — (The AIDS awareness library)
    Includes index.
    Summary: Introduces AIDS, explaining what it is, how it cannot be spread by casual contact, and how to act around someone who has it.
    ISBN 0-8239-2369-X
      1. AIDS (Disease)—Juvenile literature. [1. AIDS (Disease). 2. Diseases.] I. Title.
RC607.A26F634   1996
616.97'92—dc20   96-1507
                                                                                                                          CIP
                                                                                                                          AC

Manufactured in the United States of America

Contents

1	A Disease Called AIDS	5
2	What Causes AIDS?	6
3	Being HIV-Positive	9
4	When Someone Gets AIDS	10
5	Living with Someone with AIDS	13
6	Why Is AIDS a Big Secret?	14
7	AIDS and Staying Healthy	17
8	AIDS and Getting Sick	18
9	AIDS and Dying	21
10	You Can Help	22
	Glossary	23
	Index	24

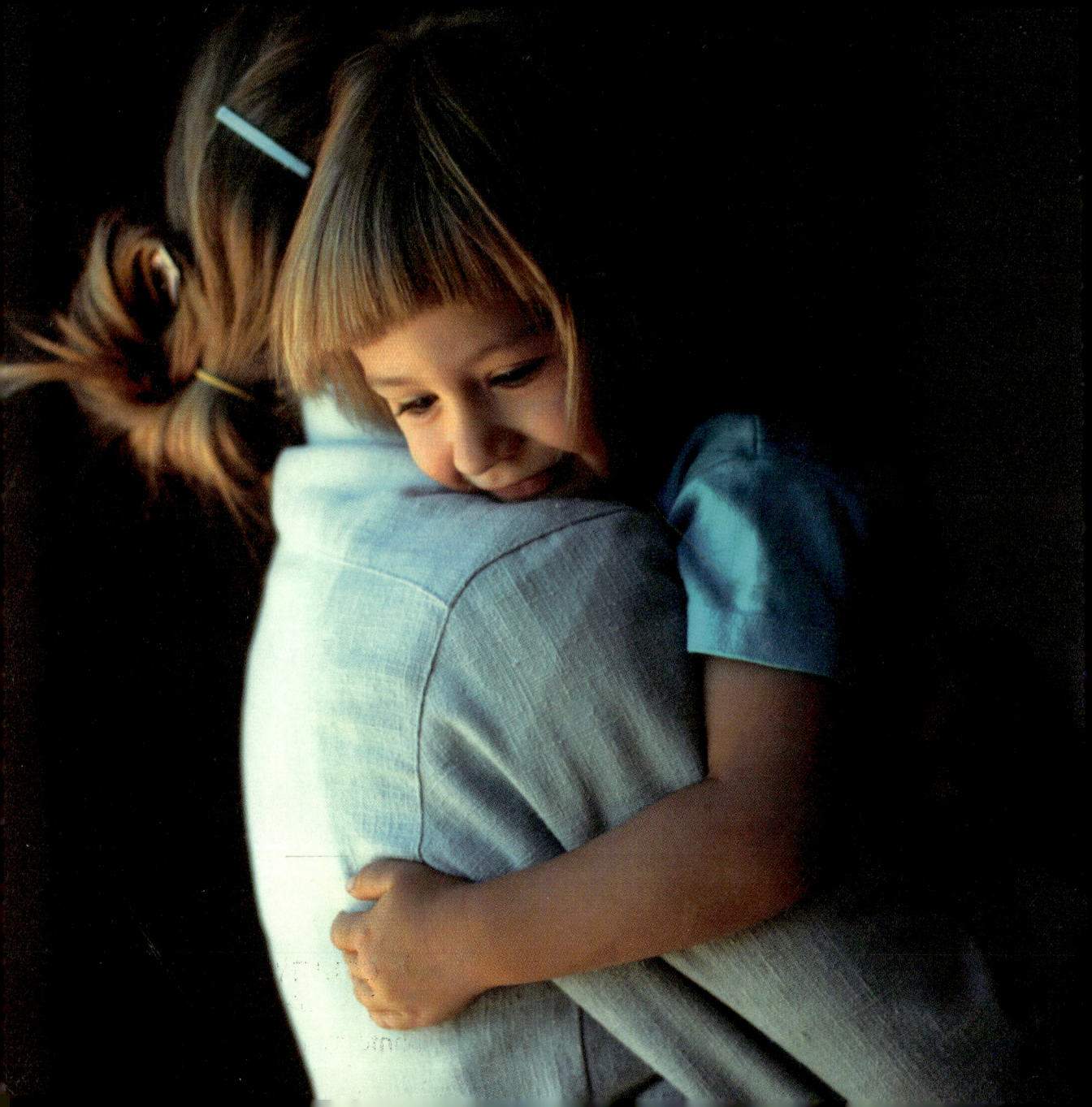

A Disease Called AIDS

This is a book about a **disease** (di-ZEEZ) called AIDS. AIDS is caused by a **virus** (VY-rus) called HIV.

About one million people in the United States have HIV. About half a million people have AIDS. You may know some of them.

This book is about what happens when someone has AIDS. It may help you deal with how it feels if someone close to you has AIDS.

◀ Diseases like AIDS can be scary and hard to understand.

What Causes AIDS?

People get AIDS from having a virus called HIV. HIV lives in someone's body for a long time before he or she gets sick. The chicken pox virus makes a person sick within two weeks. Flu germs give someone the flu within two days. But HIV doesn't usually turn into AIDS for seven to ten years after a person gets it.

People with HIV usually don't feel or look sick. ▶

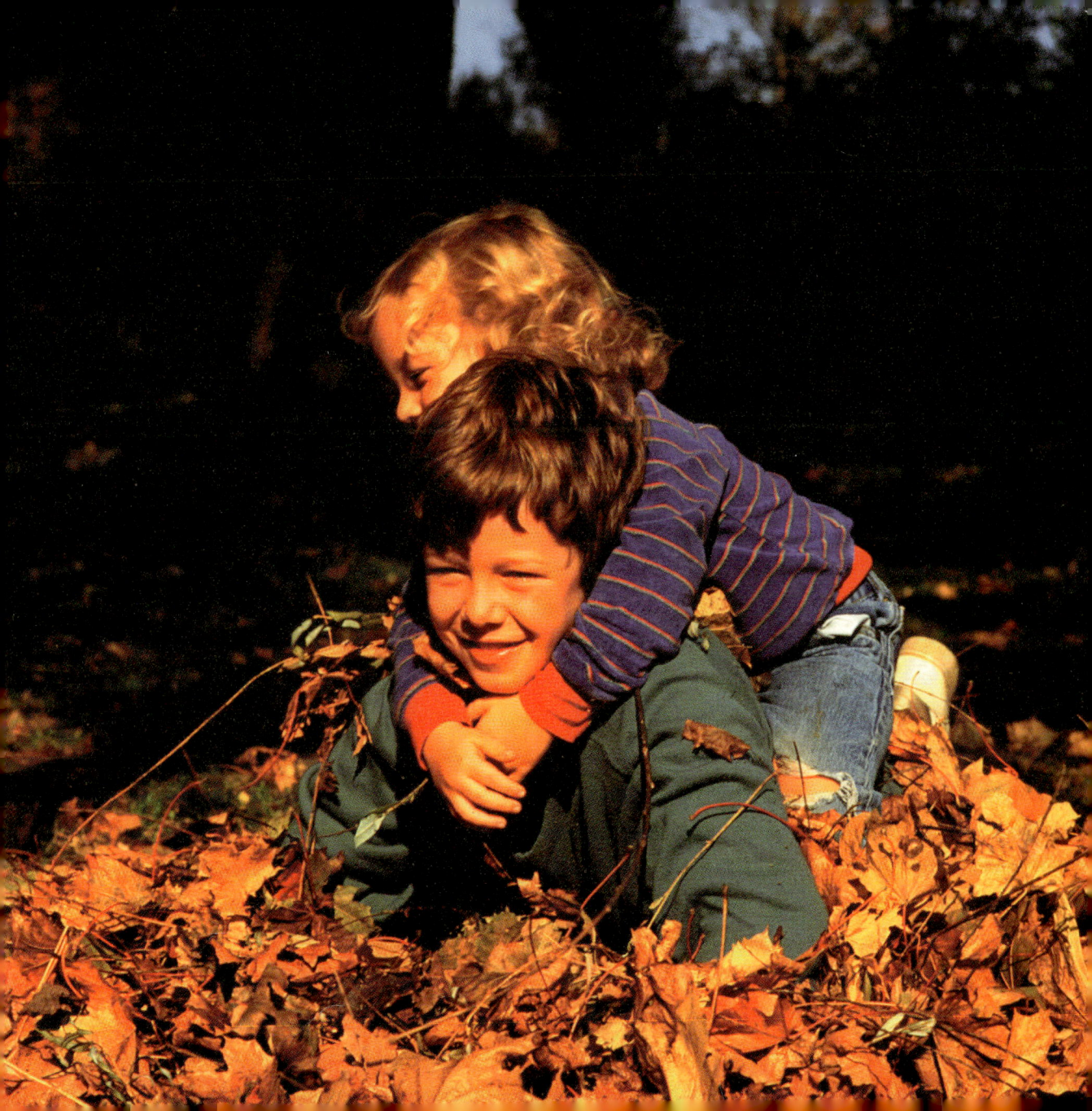

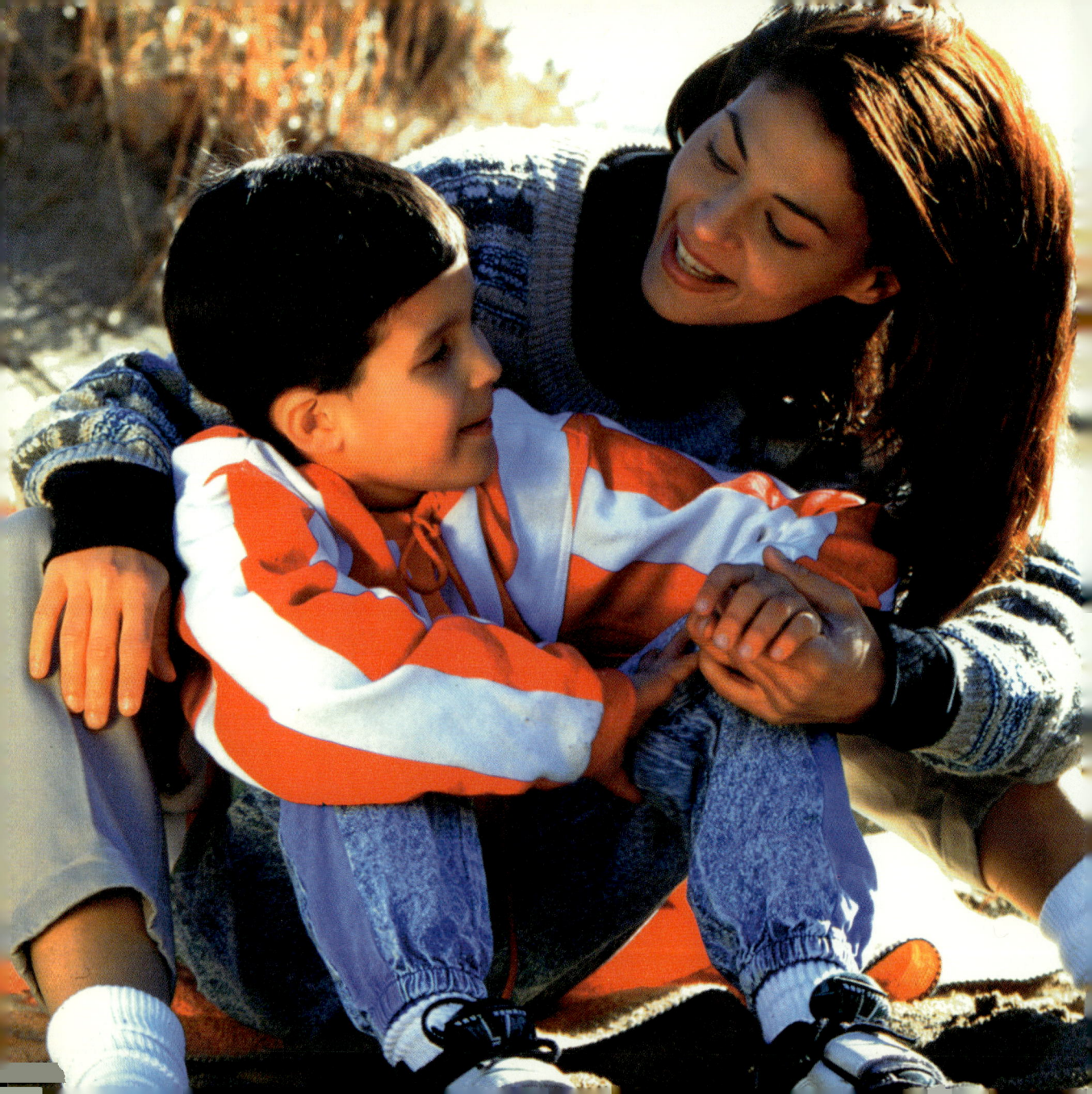

Being HIV-Positive

When people have HIV but not AIDS, we say they are **HIV-positive** (HIV POZ-i-tiv). This means that they have the virus that can cause AIDS, but they don't have AIDS. Some people have been HIV-positive for as long as fifteen years without getting AIDS.

People who are HIV-positive get AIDS when their bodies are weak and worn out from fighting HIV. This can take many years.

◀ It takes many years for a person who is HIV-positive to get AIDS.

When Someone Gets AIDS

By the time someone gets AIDS, his or her body is tired from fighting HIV. People with AIDS get so thin that, in Africa, AIDS is called the "Slim Disease."

When someone has AIDS, his body can't fight off any diseases. It gets harder and harder for him to get well when he gets sick. After a while, his body gets so weak and sick that he dies. There is no cure for AIDS yet.

A person with AIDS cannot fight off sickness.

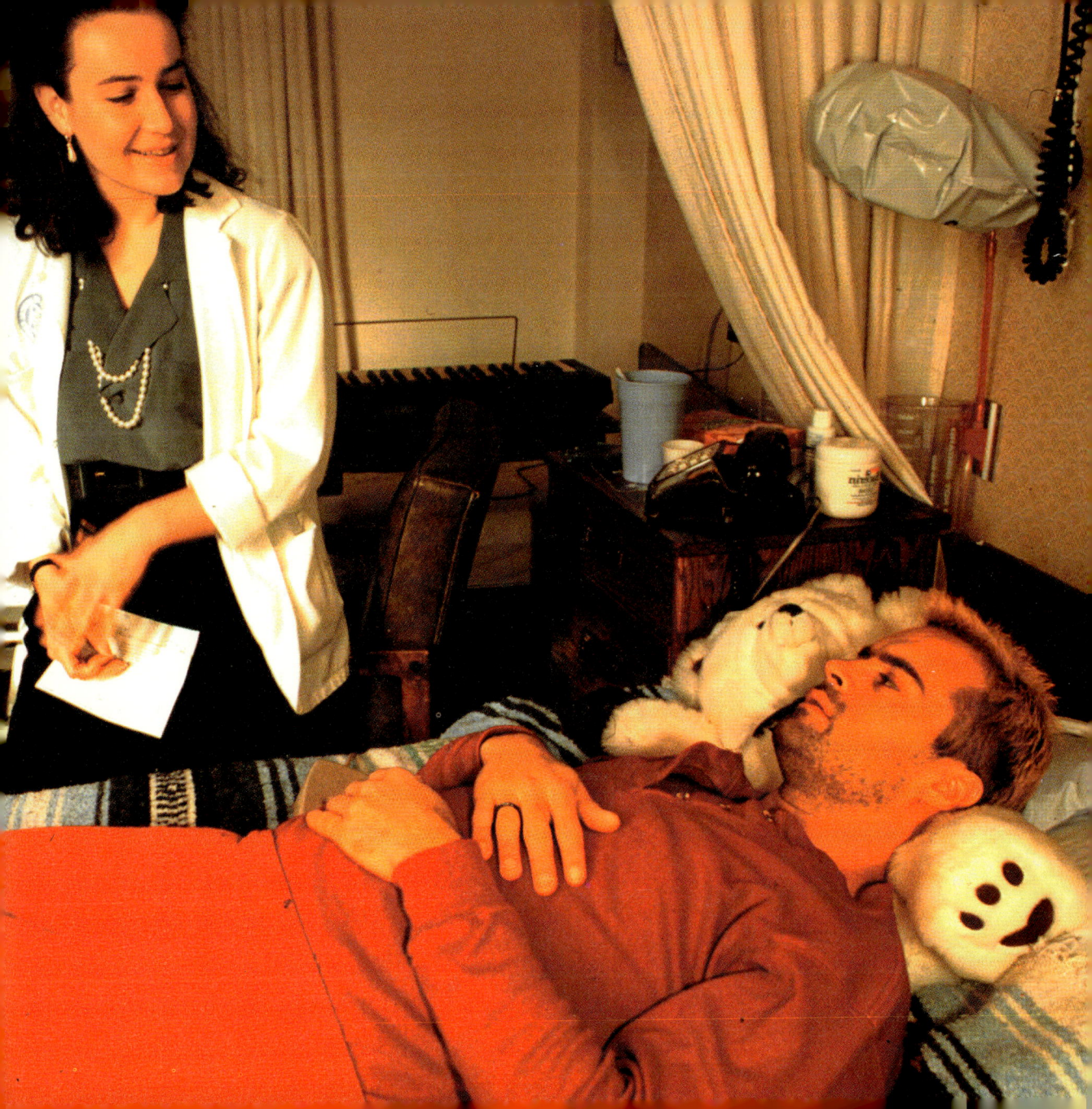

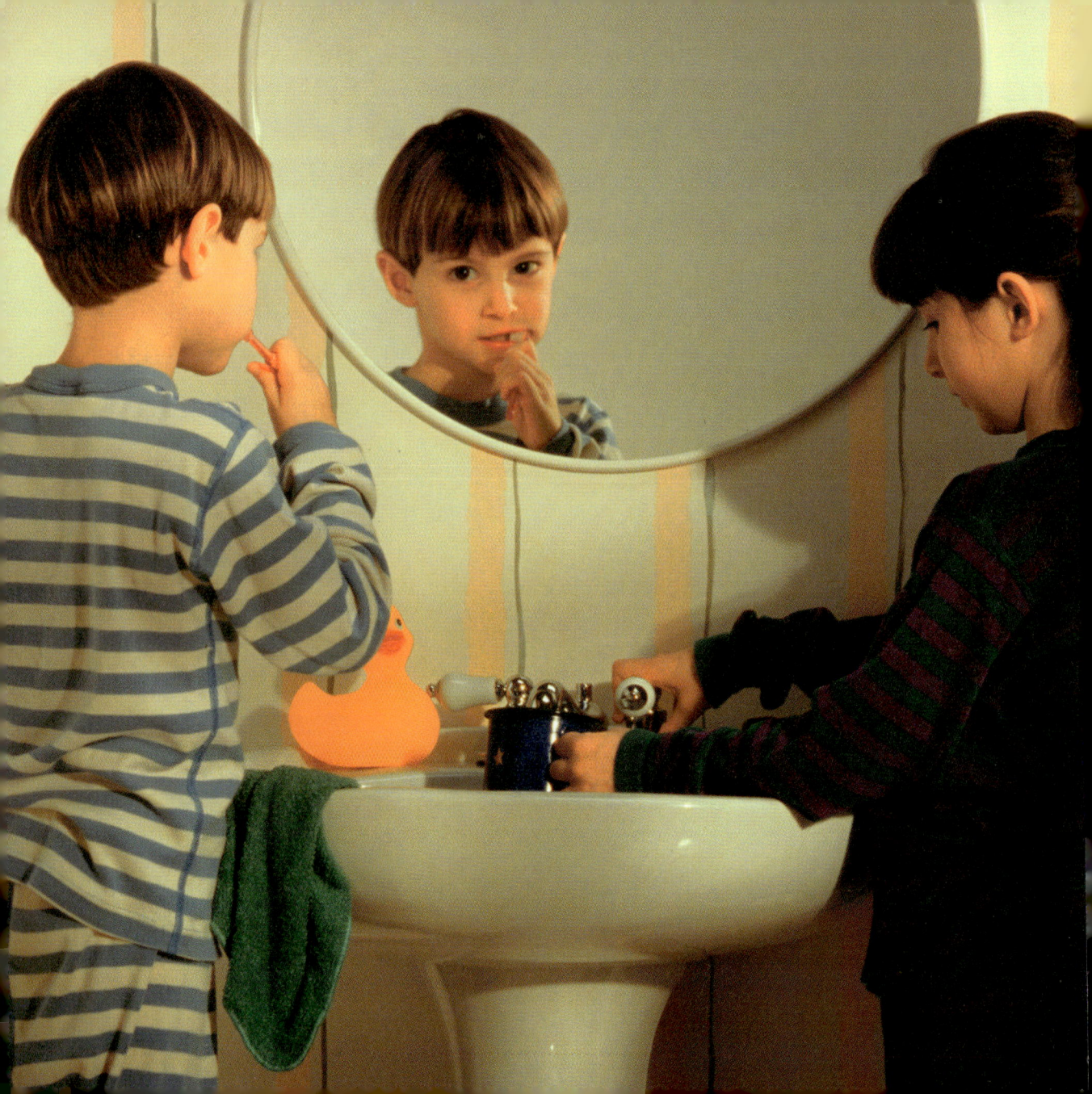

Living with Someone with AIDS

Some people are afraid to live with someone with HIV or AIDS. They may think it's easy to get HIV or AIDS from him. That's not true.

HIV and AIDS aren't spread by living together. You can't get it from hugging, or touching, or playing games or sports. You can't get it if someone with HIV or AIDS coughs or sneezes on you. Most people get HIV or AIDS by having unsafe sex or from sharing a needle when using drugs.

◀ You can't get AIDS from someone by doing everyday things with them.

Why Is AIDS a Big Secret?

Some people don't like to talk about AIDS. They're afraid of what others might think. Some people think that people with AIDS are bad. They don't want people with AIDS living in their towns or going to their schools.

But most people don't think that way. Most people know that people only get HIV by accident. It has nothing to do with what kind of people they are. Most people want to help people with HIV or AIDS.

There are many ways to show that you care about people with AIDS. ▶

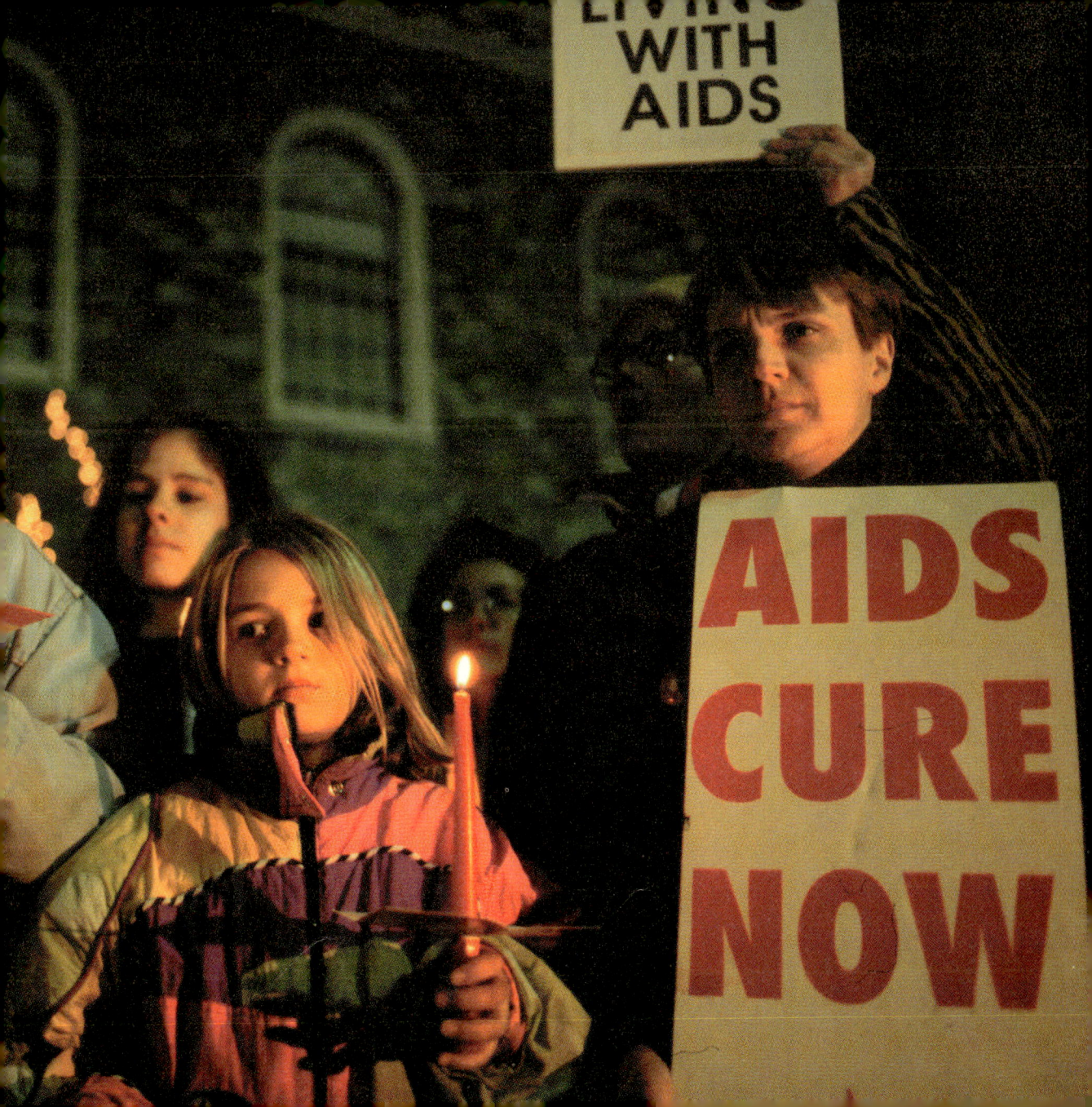

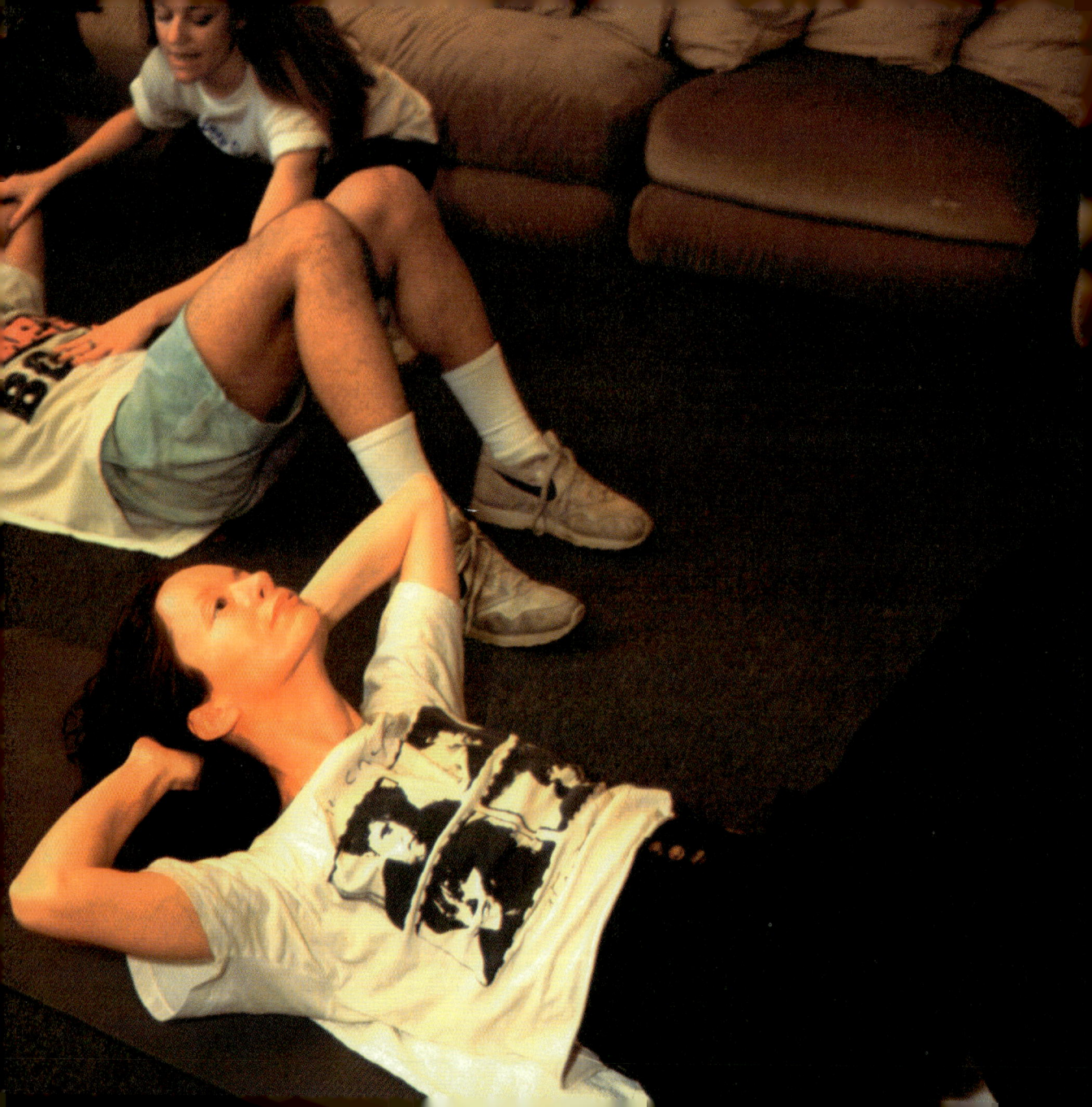

AIDS and Staying Healthy

Most people with AIDS try hard to stay healthy. They see doctors, take medicines, and get plenty of food and sleep. But AIDS is a tough disease. It knocks out a person's **immune system** (im-MYOON SIS-tem). This makes it easier to get sick, and hard to get well again. There are lots of things you can do to help a friend or relative who has AIDS. Visit her. Take her a snack that she really likes. Or just relax and keep her company.

◀ One way people with AIDS can help stay strong is by exercising.

AIDS and Getting Sick

If a person with AIDS gets very sick, friends and relatives may not be able to care for him. He might have to go to the hospital. The doctors and nurses there work hard to help people get better.

You can help someone with AIDS who is in the hospital too. You can send a funny card or a friendly note. Or call on the phone just to talk. Or tell a joke to make your friend or relative laugh. All these things help people feel better.

Sometimes people with AIDS have to stay in a hospital. ▶

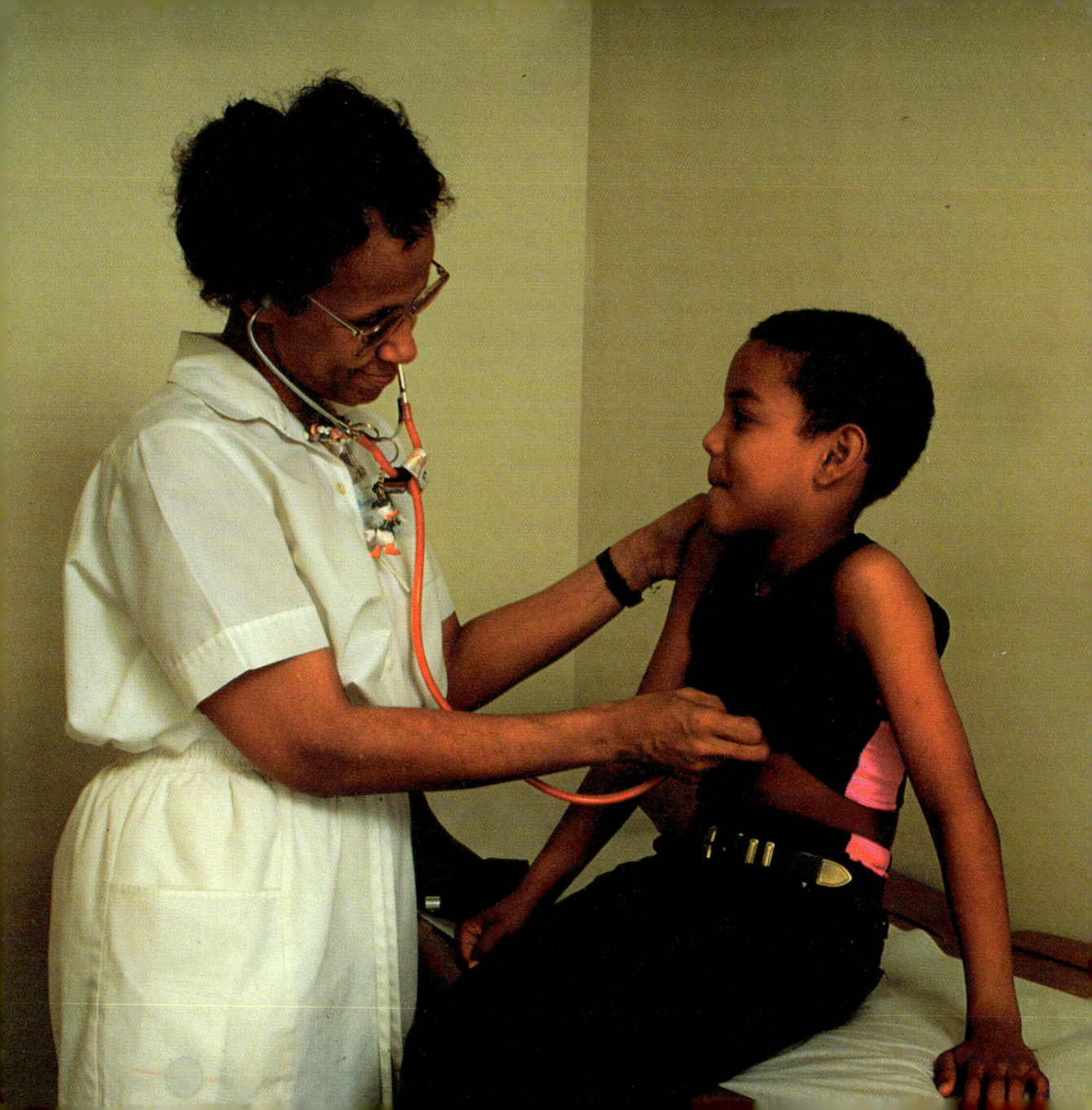

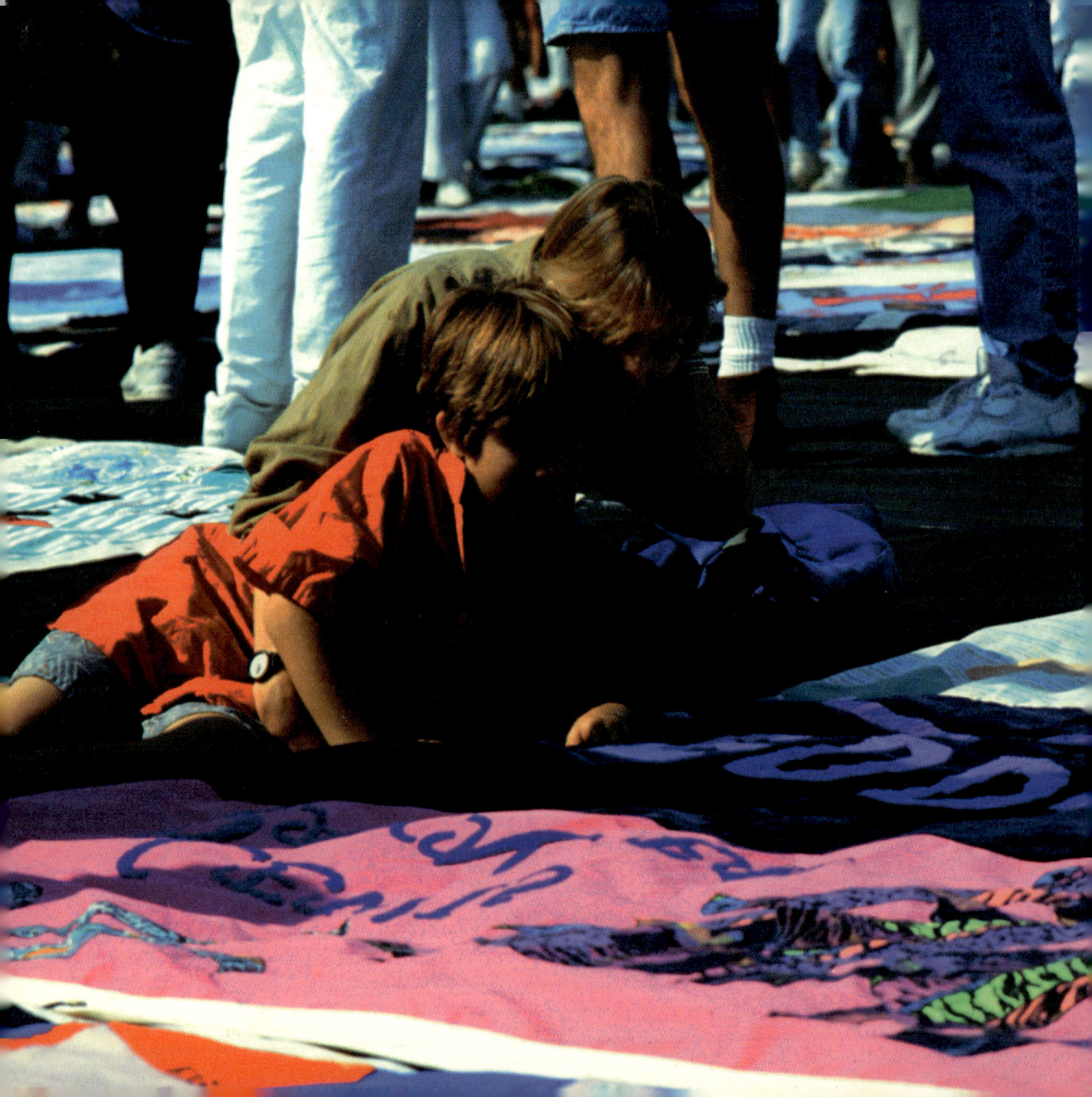

AIDS and Dying

Most of us won't die until we are very old. It's unfair, but people with AIDS die sooner than that. When someone dies, you may feel very sad or angry. These feelings are normal. Don't hold them in. Tell someone how you feel. He or she can help you feel better.

As time passes, it will be easier to think about the person who died. You'll begin to think about the happy times with that person. These **memories** (MEM-or-ees) are a way of keeping people with us.

◀ Some people remember their loved ones by making a panel for the AIDS quilt.

You Can Help

You can start helping people with AIDS by not being afraid to be around them and their families. Everybody needs friends.

When you visit with your friend or relative, remember that being sick is hard. That person may not always be happy or cheerful. But chances are, that person will be very glad you are there. Spending time with that person, bringing the latest news from school or home, and listening are the best things you can do for someone close to you who has AIDS.

LEE COUNTY LIBRARY
107 Hawkins Ave.
Sanford, NC 27330

Glossary

disease (di-ZEEZ) An illness.
HIV-positive (HIV POZ-i-tiv) Having HIV without being sick with AIDS.
immune system (im-MYOON SIS-tem) Your body's way of fighting diseases.
memories (MEM-or-ees) Things you remember about someone.
virus (VY-rus) Germ that causes illness.

Index

A
accident, 14
anger, 21

C
cure, 10

D
disease, 5, 10
dying, 21

F
friend, helping, 17, 18, 22

H
HIV, 5, 6, 9, 10, 14
  spreading of, 13
HIV-positive, 9

I
immune system, 17

L
listening, 22

M
memories, 21

S
sadness, 21
secret, 14
sickness, 18, 22
"Slim Disease," 10

V
virus, 5, 6, 9

LEE COUNTY LIBRARY SYSTEM

3 3262 00165 8977

```
J616.97
F
Forbes
When someone you know has AIDS
```

LEE COUNTY LIBRARY
107 Hawkins Ave.
Sanford, NC 27330

GAYLORD S